# Copyright (c)

# Contents

## About This Cookbook

Welcome to a culinary adventure designed exclusively for those who are passionate about sculpting their bodies and optimizing their performance. This Bodybuilding Diet Cookbook isn't just a compilation of recipes; it's your dedicated companion on the journey to achieving your fitness goals.

Tailored for Bodybuilders: This cookbook is meticulously crafted with the needs of bodybuilders and fitness enthusiasts in mind. Each recipe is a fusion of nutrition and flavor, ensuring that you don't just meet your dietary requirements but relish every bite on your path to greatness.

Nutrition Unveiled: Beyond the delectable recipes, this cookbook unveils the science behind nutrition. Dive into the principles of macronutrients, learn about strategic meal planning, and discover the role of supplements in maximizing your results. We believe that knowledge is power, and with the right information, you can elevate your nutrition game.

Balancing Taste and Performance: Gone are the days of compromising taste for fitness. Here, you'll discover a harmonious blend of flavors and functionality. From savory main courses to tempting desserts, each dish is a testament to the idea that eating for performance can be a delight for the taste buds.

Versatility for All Levels: Whether you're a seasoned bodybuilder or just starting your fitness journey, this cookbook caters to all levels of expertise. Find inspiration for every meal, snack, and treat, ensuring that your nutrition aligns seamlessly with your goals.

A Culinary Blueprint: Consider this cookbook your culinary blueprint for success. With detailed nutritional insights, sample meal plans, and practical tips, we guide you through transforming your kitchen into a hub for muscle-building, energy-boosting, and performance-enhancing creations.

Embark on this flavorful and nourishing journey with us. The kitchen is your training ground, and each recipe is a step towards your peak performance. Get ready to savor the taste of success – because your body deserves nothing less.


The Importance of Nutrition in Bodybuilding

Embarking on the path of bodybuilding demands more than just rigorous workouts and heavy lifting. The cornerstone of a successful and sustainable bodybuilding journey is, without a doubt, nutrition. It's not just about the quantity of food you consume but the quality and strategic balance that fuel your body towards optimal performance and growth.

Fueling the Machine: Think of your body as a high-performance machine. To push it to its limits and ensure it functions at its best, you need the right fuel. Nutrition provides the raw materials needed for muscle repair, growth, and overall recovery. Each meal is an opportunity to replenish glycogen stores, repair microtears in muscle fibers, and supply the body with essential nutrients for peak functioning.

Building Blocks of Muscle: Proteins, the building blocks of muscles, take center stage in a bodybuilder's diet. Adequate protein intake is crucial for muscle protein synthesis, the process that repairs and builds new muscle tissue. A well-balanced diet ensures that your body has the amino acids necessary for this continuous rebuilding process.

Energy for Intense Workouts: Carbohydrates are the body's primary source of energy. For bodybuilders engaging in high-intensity workouts, a sufficient intake of complex carbohydrates is essential. These carbs provide the energy needed to power through demanding training sessions, supporting both strength and endurance.

Fat for Hormonal Balance: While often misunderstood, fats play a crucial role in hormonal balance. Hormones such as testosterone, growth hormone, and insulin, which are vital for muscle growth, rely on a healthy fat intake. Including the right types of fats in your diet is fundamental for sustaining energy levels and promoting overall well-being.

Optimizing Recovery: The post-workout period is when your body is primed for recovery and growth. Nutrition during this window is critical. Properly timed meals with the right blend of nutrients - proteins, carbohydrates, and fats - can enhance recovery, reduce muscle soreness, and set the stage for your next training session.

Strategic Meal Planning: Bodybuilding nutrition isn't just about individual meals; it's about the bigger picture. Strategic meal planning ensures a steady and balanced supply of nutrients throughout the day, optimizing your body's ability to build and maintain muscle mass.

In this journey of sculpting your physique, remember that what you eat is as important as how you train. The right nutrition plan isn't a mere complement to your workouts; it's the foundation upon which your bodybuilding success is built. So, let's delve into the art and science of nourishing your body for unparalleled results. Your transformation begins with what's on your plate.

## How to Use This Cookbook

Congratulations on taking the first step towards a culinary and fitness adventure with our Bodybuilding Diet Cookbook. To make the most of this resource and seamlessly integrate it into your lifestyle, follow these guidelines:

1. Introduction: Familiarize yourself with the introductory section. Understand the philosophy behind the cookbook, its target audience, and the unique approach to nutrition for bodybuilding. This will set the tone for your journey.

2. Understanding Macronutrients: Dive into the section on macronutrients. Learn about the role of proteins, carbohydrates, and fats in your bodybuilding journey. Gain insights into the importance of each macronutrient, optimal intake levels, and their strategic placement in your diet.

3. Meal Planning Basics: Discover the fundamentals of meal planning. Understand how to calculate your daily caloric needs, portion control, and the timing of meals for pre- and post-workout nutrition. This section lays the groundwork for structuring your daily food intake.

4. Recipes Galore: The heart of the cookbook lies in its diverse and delicious recipes. Explore the breakfast, lunch, dinner, snack, and dessert sections. Each recipe is designed to offer a perfect blend of taste and

nutrition. Feel free to experiment, mix and match, and find your favorite go-to meals.

5. Nutrition for Muscle Building and Fat Loss: Delve deeper into the science of nutrition for body composition goals. Learn about the role of supplements, timing your meals for optimal results, and how to adjust your nutrition during bulking and cutting phases.

6. Sample Meal Plans: Take advantage of the sample meal plans provided. These are practical guides to help you structure your daily and weekly meals based on your goals. Whether you're a beginner or an advanced bodybuilder, these plans offer a roadmap for success.

7. Tips for Success: Explore the tips section for valuable insights on grocery shopping, meal prep, and maintaining consistency with your diet. These practical tips will help you seamlessly incorporate the principles of this cookbook into your daily routine.

8. Conclusion: Wrap up your exploration with the concluding section. Reflect on the insights gained, acknowledge your commitment to your nutritional journey, and find motivation to carry the principles forward.

Remember, this cookbook is not just a collection of recipes but a comprehensive guide to transforming your approach to nutrition. Get ready to savor delicious meals while fueling your body for success. Your journey towards a stronger, healthier you starts now. Enjoy the process!

# A 14-day Meal Plan

Day 1:

Breakfast: Protein-Packed Smoothie Bowl

1. Blend together frozen berries, a banana, Greek yogurt, and protein powder.

2. Pour the smoothie into a bowl.

3. Top with granola, sliced almonds, and a drizzle of honey.

Lunch: Grilled Chicken Salad

1. Grill chicken breast slices.

2. Mix grilled chicken with salad greens, cherry tomatoes, and cucumber.

3. Drizzle with balsamic vinaigrette.

Snack: Hummus with Veggie Sticks

1. Dip carrot sticks, cucumber slices, and bell pepper strips into hummus.

Dinner: Lentil and Sweet Potato Curry

1. Cook lentils and sweet potatoes in a curry-spiced coconut milk broth.

Day 2:

Breakfast: Scrambled Eggs with Vegetables

1. Sauté chopped vegetables (bell peppers, onions, spinach) in a pan.

2. Beat eggs and pour over the vegetables, stirring until fully cooked.

Lunch: Turkey and Quinoa Stuffed Peppers

1. Brown ground turkey in a skillet, mix with cooked quinoa.

2. Stuff bell peppers with the turkey-quinoa mixture, top with tomato sauce and cheese.

3. Bake until peppers are tender.

Snack: Hard-Boiled Eggs with Sriracha

1. Slice hard-boiled eggs and drizzle with Sriracha sauce.

Dinner: Chickpea and Spinach Stir-Fry

1. Sauté chickpeas, fresh spinach, and minced garlic in a pan with soy sauce.

Day 3:

Breakfast: Greek Yogurt Parfait

1. Layer Greek yogurt, granola, and mixed berries in a glass or bowl.

2. Repeat the layers and drizzle with honey.

Lunch: Quinoa Salad with Chickpeas

1. Mix cooked quinoa with chickpeas, cherry tomatoes, cucumber, and feta cheese.

Snack: Cottage Cheese Pancakes

1. Blend cottage cheese, eggs, oat flour, and vanilla extract until smooth.

2. Cook small portions of batter in a skillet to make pancakes.

Dinner: Grilled Lean Steak with Sweet Potato Mash

1. Grill lean steak to your liking.

2. Mash sweet potatoes and serve alongside the grilled steak with asparagus spears.

Day 4:

Breakfast: Chia Seed Pudding

1. Mix chia seeds, almond milk, and vanilla extract in a jar.

2. Refrigerate overnight.

3. Top with fresh fruit before serving.

Lunch: Spinach and Feta Omelette

1. Whisk eggs in a bowl and season with salt and pepper.

2. Sauté chopped spinach until wilted, then pour whisked eggs over it.

3. Add feta cheese and cook until set.

Snack: Almond Butter and Banana Toast

1. Toast slices of whole-grain bread.

2. Spread almond butter on the toast and top with banana slices.

Dinner: Quinoa Porridge

1. Cook quinoa with almond milk until it reaches a porridge-like consistency.

2. Top with sliced almonds, berries, and a drizzle of honey.

Day 5:

Breakfast: Protein Smoothie with Banana, Spinach, and Almond Milk

1. Blend one banana, a handful of spinach, a scoop of protein powder, and almond milk until smooth.

Lunch: Grilled Chicken Wrap

1. Grill chicken strips and place them in a whole-grain tortilla.

2. Add lettuce, tomatoes, and a drizzle of Greek yogurt as a dressing.

3. Roll the tortilla into a wrap.

Snack: Mixed Nuts

1. Grab a handful of mixed nuts for a quick and protein-packed snack.

Dinner: Baked Salmon with Quinoa

1. Season salmon fillets with herbs and lemon.

2. Bake until it flakes easily with a fork.

3. Serve over a bed of cooked quinoa and steamed broccoli.

Day 6:

Breakfast: Oatmeal topped with Sliced Banana and Chia Seeds

1. Cook oats according to package instructions.

2. Top with sliced banana and a sprinkle of chia seeds.

Lunch: Lentil and Vegetable Stir-Fry

1. Sauté lentils with mixed vegetables (bell peppers, broccoli, carrots) in soy sauce.

2. Serve over brown rice.

Snack: Apple Slices with Almond Butter

1. Slice an apple into wedges.

2. Spread almond butter on each apple slice.

Dinner: Stir-Fried Tofu with Brown Rice

1. Sauté tofu and assorted vegetables in a pan with teriyaki sauce.

2. Serve over cooked brown rice.

Day 7:

Breakfast: Blueberry Protein Pancakes

1. Mix protein powder, oat flour, and blueberries.

2. Cook small portions on a skillet to make pancakes.

3. Top with Greek yogurt and a drizzle of honey.

Lunch: Shrimp and Quinoa Salad

1. Sauté shrimp with garlic and lemon juice.

2. Mix with cooked quinoa, cherry tomatoes, and arugula.

3. Dress with olive oil and lemon vinaigrette.

Snack: Chocolate Protein Smoothie

1. Blend almond milk, protein powder, a banana, and a tablespoon of cocoa powder.

Dinner: Baked Cod with Sweet Potato Fries

1. Season cod fillets with herbs and lemon.

2. Bake until cooked through.

3. Serve with baked sweet potato fries.

Day 8:

Breakfast: Peanut Butter Banana Overnight Oats

1. Mix rolled oats, almond milk, sliced bananas, and a spoonful of peanut butter.

2. Refrigerate overnight.

Lunch: Turkey and Avocado Salad Wrap

1. Lay a whole-grain tortilla flat.

2. Fill with sliced turkey, avocado, lettuce, and cherry tomatoes.

3. Roll into a wrap.

Snack: Cottage Cheese with Pineapple Chunks

1. Combine cottage cheese with fresh pineapple chunks.

Dinner: Beef and Broccoli Stir-Fry

1. Stir-fry lean beef strips with broccoli and garlic in soy sauce.

2. Serve over brown rice.

Day 9:

Breakfast: Mango Protein Smoothie Bowl

1. Blend frozen mango, protein powder, and almond milk.

2. Pour into a bowl and top with granola and sliced almonds.

Lunch: Caprese Quinoa Salad

1. Mix cooked quinoa with cherry tomatoes, fresh mozzarella, and basil.

2. Drizzle with balsamic glaze.

Snack: Rice Cake with Almond Butter

1. Spread almond butter on a rice cake for a quick and satisfying snack.

Dinner: Grilled Vegetable and Chickpea Bowl

1. Grill zucchini, bell peppers, and eggplant.

2. Combine with chickpeas and quinoa.

3. Drizzle with tahini dressing.

Day 10:

Breakfast: Raspberry Chia Seed Pudding

1. Mix chia seeds with almond milk, raspberries, and a touch of honey.

2. Refrigerate overnight.

Lunch: Chicken and Quinoa Stuffed Bell Peppers

1. Cook quinoa and mix with shredded chicken.

2. Stuff bell peppers with the quinoa-chicken mixture.

3. Bake until peppers are tender.

Snack: Celery Sticks with Hummus

1. Dip celery sticks into hummus for a satisfying and crunchy snack.

Dinner: Turkey and Vegetable Skewers

1. Thread turkey cubes, cherry tomatoes, and bell peppers onto skewers.

2. Grill until turkey is cooked and veggies are charred.

Day 11:

Breakfast: Spinach and Feta Egg Muffins

1. Whisk eggs and mix with chopped spinach and feta cheese.

2. Pour into muffin cups and bake until set.

Lunch: Quinoa and Black Bean Bowl

1. Combine cooked quinoa, black beans, corn, and diced tomatoes.

2. Top with avocado slices and a squeeze of lime.

Snack: Greek Yogurt with Berries

1. Mix Greek yogurt with fresh berries for a creamy and fruity snack.

Dinner: Teriyaki Salmon with Steamed Broccoli

1. Marinate salmon fillets in teriyaki sauce.

2. Bake until the salmon flakes easily.

3. Serve with steamed broccoli.

Day 12:

Breakfast: Apple Cinnamon Protein Oatmeal

1. Cook oats with almond milk, diced apples, and a sprinkle of cinnamon.

2. Stir in your favorite protein powder.

Lunch: Chickpea and Avocado Wrap

1. Mash chickpeas with avocado, lime juice, and cilantro.

2. Spread the mixture onto a whole-grain tortilla and roll it up.

Snack: Trail Mix with Dark Chocolate

1. Create a trail mix with mixed nuts, dried fruits, and dark chocolate chunks.

Dinner: Baked Chicken Thighs with Roasted Brussels Sprouts

1. Season chicken thighs with herbs and bake until golden.

2. Roast Brussels sprouts with olive oil, salt, and pepper.

Day 13:

Breakfast: Banana Walnut Protein Muffins

1. Mix mashed bananas, protein powder, and chopped walnuts.

2. Bake in muffin cups until cooked through.

Lunch: Shrimp and Asparagus Stir-Fry

1. Sauté shrimp and asparagus in a pan with garlic and soy sauce.

2. Serve over brown rice.

Snack: Cottage Cheese with Tomatoes and Basil

1. Combine cottage cheese with cherry tomatoes and fresh basil.

Dinner: Quinoa and Vegetable Stuffed Portobello Mushrooms

1. Mix cooked quinoa with diced vegetables.

2. Stuff portobello mushrooms and bake until tender.

Day 14:

Breakfast: Blueberry Almond Butter Protein Smoothie

1. Blend almond milk, blueberries, almond butter, and protein powder.

Lunch: Turkey and Spinach Wrap

1. Layer sliced turkey, spinach, and hummus onto a whole-grain tortilla.

2. Roll it up and enjoy.

Snack: Rice Cake with Cottage Cheese and Pineapple

1. Spread cottage cheese on a rice cake and top with pineapple chunks.

Dinner: Grilled Tofu with Quinoa Salad

1. Grill tofu slices marinated in your favorite sauce.

2. Serve over a quinoa salad with mixed veggies.

Day 15:

Breakfast: Peanut Butter Banana Protein Waffles

1. Prepare waffle batter with protein powder, mashed bananas, and peanut butter.

2. Cook in a waffle iron until golden.

Lunch: Spinach and Chickpea Salad with Feta

1. Toss fresh spinach with chickpeas, cherry tomatoes, and crumbled feta cheese.

2. Dress with olive oil and balsamic vinegar.

Snack: Greek Yogurt Parfait with Mango

1. Layer Greek yogurt with diced mango and a sprinkle of granola.

Dinner: Baked Cod with Lemon Dill Sauce

1. Season cod fillets with lemon, dill, and a touch of olive oil.

2. Bake until the fish is flaky.

Day 16:

Breakfast: Chocolate Avocado Protein Smoothie

1. Blend almond milk, protein powder, ripe avocado, and a tablespoon of cocoa powder.

Lunch: Quinoa and Vegetable Wrap

1. Fill a whole-grain wrap with cooked quinoa, sautéed vegetables, and a drizzle of tahini.

Snack: Cottage Cheese with Berries and Almonds

1. Mix cottage cheese with fresh berries and a handful of almonds.

Dinner: Teriyaki Beef Stir-Fry

1. Stir-fry lean beef strips with broccoli, bell peppers, and snap peas in teriyaki sauce.

2. Serve over a bed of brown rice.

Day 17:

Breakfast: Blueberry Protein Pancake Stack

1. Make a stack of protein pancakes using blueberries in the batter.

2. Top with Greek yogurt and a sprinkle of cinnamon.

Lunch: Mediterranean Chickpea Salad

1. Combine chickpeas, cucumber, cherry tomatoes, olives, and feta.

2. Dress with olive oil, lemon juice, and oregano.

Snack: Rice Cake with Hummus and Sliced Cucumber

1. Spread hummus on a rice cake and top with cucumber slices.

Dinner: Salmon and Asparagus Foil Pack

1. Place salmon fillets and asparagus spears on a sheet of foil.

2. Season with lemon, dill, and fold into a sealed packet before baking.

Day 18:

Breakfast: Raspberry Almond Protein Muffins

1. Mix protein powder, almond flour, and fresh raspberries.

2. Bake in muffin cups until cooked through.

Lunch: Turkey and Quinoa Bowl

1. Combine ground turkey with cooked quinoa, black beans, corn, and salsa.

Snack: Apple Slices with Peanut Butter

1. Slice an apple and enjoy with a dollop of peanut butter.

Dinner: Grilled Chicken Caesar Salad

1. Grill chicken breast and slice.

2. Toss with romaine lettuce, cherry tomatoes, croutons, and Caesar dressing.

Day 19:

Breakfast: Mango Coconut Chia Pudding

1. Mix chia seeds with coconut milk, diced mango, and a touch of honey.

2. Refrigerate until set.

Lunch: Tuna and Avocado Lettuce Wraps

1. Mix canned tuna with diced avocado, red onion, and cilantro.

2. Serve in lettuce wraps.

Snack: Greek Yogurt with Pistachios

1. Top Greek yogurt with crushed pistachios for a satisfying crunch.

Dinner: Vegetable and Lentil Curry

1. Cook lentils with a variety of vegetables in a coconut milk and curry sauce.

**Certainly! Here are five high-protein breakfast recipes with step-by-step instructions and ingredients:**

1. Protein-Packed Smoothie Bowl:

Ingredients:

• 1 cup frozen mixed berries

• 1 banana

• 1 cup Greek yogurt

• 1 scoop protein powder

• Toppings: Granola, sliced almonds, honey

Instructions:

1. In a blender, combine frozen berries, banana, Greek yogurt, and protein powder.

2. Blend until smooth.

3. Pour the smoothie into a bowl.

4. Top with granola, sliced almonds, and a drizzle of honey.

2. Scrambled Eggs with Vegetables:

Ingredients:

• 3 large eggs

• 1/2 cup diced bell peppers

• 1/2 cup diced tomatoes

• 1/4 cup diced onions

• Salt and pepper to taste

• Cooking spray or olive oil

Instructions:

1. In a bowl, beat the eggs and season with salt and pepper.

2. Heat a pan over medium heat and add cooking spray or olive oil.

3. Sauté diced bell peppers, tomatoes, and onions until softened.

4. Pour beaten eggs over the vegetables and scramble until cooked through.

3. Overnight Oats with Berries:

Ingredients:

• 1/2 cup rolled oats

• 1/2 cup Greek yogurt

- 1/2 cup almond milk

- 1 tablespoon chia seeds

- Mixed berries for topping

Instructions:

1. In a jar, mix rolled oats, Greek yogurt, almond milk, and chia seeds.

2. Stir well, cover, and refrigerate overnight.

3. In the morning, top with mixed berries before serving.

4. Quinoa Porridge:

Ingredients:

- 1/2 cup cooked quinoa

- 1/2 cup almond milk

- 1 tablespoon almond butter

- Sliced banana and chopped nuts for topping

Instructions:

1. In a saucepan, heat cooked quinoa and almond milk.

2. Stir in almond butter until well combined.

3. Simmer until the mixture thickens.

4. Pour into a bowl and top with sliced banana and chopped nuts.

5. Greek Yogurt Parfait:

Ingredients:

• 1 cup Greek yogurt

• 1/2 cup granola

• 1/2 cup mixed berries

• 1 tablespoon honey

Instructions:

1. In a glass or bowl, layer Greek yogurt, granola, and mixed berries.

2. Repeat the layers.

3. Drizzle honey on top.


**Certainly! Here are five protein-packed smoothie bowl recipes with step-by-step instructions and ingredients:**

1. Berry Blast Protein Smoothie Bowl:

Ingredients:

• 1 cup frozen mixed berries (strawberries, blueberries, raspberries)

• 1 banana

• 1/2 cup Greek yogurt

• 1 scoop protein powder (vanilla or berry-flavored)

• Toppings: Granola, sliced almonds, chia seeds

Instructions:

1. In a blender, combine frozen berries, banana, Greek yogurt, and protein powder.

2. Blend until smooth.

3. Pour the smoothie into a bowl.

4. Top with granola, sliced almonds, and a sprinkle of chia seeds.

2. Tropical Paradise Protein Smoothie Bowl:

Ingredients:

• 1 cup frozen pineapple chunks

• 1/2 frozen banana

• 1/2 cup Greek yogurt

• 1 scoop protein powder (vanilla or tropical-flavored)

• Toppings: Coconut flakes, sliced kiwi, chopped mango

Instructions:

1. Blend frozen pineapple, banana, Greek yogurt, and protein powder until smooth.

2. Transfer the smoothie to a bowl.

3. Top with coconut flakes, sliced kiwi, and chopped mango.

3. Chocolate Peanut Butter Protein Smoothie Bowl:

Ingredients:

• 1 cup almond milk

• 1 scoop chocolate protein powder

• 1 tablespoon peanut butter

• 1 frozen banana

• Toppings: Sliced strawberries, crushed nuts, dark chocolate shavings

Instructions:

1. Blend almond milk, chocolate protein powder, peanut butter, and frozen banana until creamy.

2. Pour the smoothie into a bowl.

3. Top with sliced strawberries, crushed nuts, and dark chocolate shavings.

4. Green Goddess Protein Smoothie Bowl:

Ingredients:

• 1 cup spinach leaves

• 1/2 avocado

• 1/2 cup Greek yogurt

• 1 scoop protein powder (vanilla or unflavored)

• Toppings: Sliced kiwi, hemp seeds, pumpkin seeds

Instructions:

1. Blend spinach, avocado, Greek yogurt, and protein powder until smooth.

2. Transfer the green smoothie to a bowl.

3. Top with sliced kiwi, hemp seeds, and pumpkin seeds.

5. Coffee Lover's Protein Smoothie Bowl:

Ingredients:

• 1/2 cup brewed and chilled coffee

• 1/2 cup almond milk

• 1 scoop mocha or coffee-flavored protein powder

• 1 frozen banana

• Toppings: Granola, cacao nibs, sliced banana

Instructions:

1. Blend coffee, almond milk, coffee-flavored protein powder, and frozen banana until smooth.

2. Pour the coffee-infused smoothie into a bowl.

3. Top with granola, cacao nibs, and sliced banana.

Feel free to customize these smoothie bowls with your favorite protein powder flavors and toppings. Adjust the quantities to meet your nutritional needs and taste preferences. Enjoy your protein-packed and delicious smoothie bowls!

**Certainly! Here are five variations of scrambled eggs with vegetables, each with its unique twist:**

1. Classic Veggie Scramble:

Ingredients:

• 3 large eggs

• 1/4 cup diced bell peppers (red, green, or both)

- 1/4 cup diced tomatoes

- 1/4 cup diced onions

- Salt and pepper to taste

- Fresh herbs (optional, for garnish)

Instructions:

1. In a bowl, whisk the eggs and season with salt and pepper.

2. Heat a non-stick pan over medium heat.

3. Sauté diced bell peppers, tomatoes, and onions until softened.

4. Pour the beaten eggs over the vegetables.

5. Gently scramble the eggs until fully cooked.

6. Garnish with fresh herbs if desired.

2. Spinach and Feta Scramble:

Ingredients:

- 3 large eggs

- 1 cup fresh spinach, chopped

- 2 tablespoons crumbled feta cheese

- Salt and pepper to taste

• Olive oil for cooking

Instructions:

1. Whisk the eggs in a bowl and season with salt and pepper.

2. Heat olive oil in a pan over medium heat.

3. Add chopped spinach and sauté until wilted.

4. Pour the beaten eggs over the spinach.

5. Sprinkle crumbled feta over the eggs.

6. Scramble until the eggs are fully cooked.

3. Mushroom and Onion Scramble:

Ingredients:

• 3 large eggs

• 1/2 cup sliced mushrooms

• 1/4 cup diced onions

• Salt and pepper to taste

• Fresh parsley (optional, for garnish)

Instructions:

1. Beat the eggs in a bowl and season with salt and pepper.

2. In a pan, sauté sliced mushrooms and diced onions until golden.

3. Pour the beaten eggs over the mushrooms and onions.

4. Scramble until the eggs are cooked to your liking.

5. Garnish with fresh parsley if desired.

4. Tomato and Basil Scramble:

Ingredients:

• 3 large eggs

• 1/2 cup cherry tomatoes, halved

• Fresh basil leaves, chopped

• Salt and pepper to taste

• Olive oil for cooking

Instructions:

1. Whisk the eggs in a bowl and season with salt and pepper.

2. Heat olive oil in a pan over medium heat.

3. Add cherry tomatoes and sauté briefly.

4. Pour the beaten eggs over the tomatoes.

5. Sprinkle chopped basil over the eggs.

6. Scramble until the eggs are fully cooked.

5. Mediterranean Veggie Scramble:

Ingredients:

• 3 large eggs

• 1/4 cup diced red bell pepper

• 1/4 cup diced cucumber

• 2 tablespoons sliced black olives

• Feta cheese crumbles

• Salt and pepper to taste

Instructions:

1. Beat the eggs in a bowl and season with salt and pepper.

2. In a pan, sauté diced red bell pepper until softened.

3. Add diced cucumber and sliced black olives, sauté for a few minutes.

4. Pour the beaten eggs over the vegetables.

5. Sprinkle feta cheese crumbles over the eggs.

6. Scramble until the eggs are cooked through.

Certainly! Here are five energizing oatmeal variations, each with its unique flavors and ingredients:

1. Overnight Oats with Berries:

Ingredients:

• 1/2 cup rolled oats

• 1/2 cup milk (dairy or plant-based)

• 1/2 cup mixed berries (strawberries, blueberries, raspberries)

• 1 tablespoon chia seeds

• 1 teaspoon honey or maple syrup

• Almond slices for topping

Instructions:

1. In a jar, combine rolled oats, milk, mixed berries, chia seeds, and sweetener.

2. Stir well, cover, and refrigerate overnight.

3. In the morning, top with almond slices before serving.

2. Quinoa Porridge with Banana and Almonds:

Ingredients:

• 1/2 cup cooked quinoa

- 1/2 cup almond milk

- 1 ripe banana, mashed

- 1 tablespoon almond butter

- Chopped almonds for topping

- Cinnamon for garnish

Instructions:

1. In a saucepan, heat cooked quinoa and almond milk.

2. Stir in mashed banana and almond butter.

3. Simmer until the mixture thickens.

4. Pour into a bowl, top with chopped almonds, and sprinkle with cinnamon.

3. Apple Cinnamon Oatmeal:

Ingredients:

- 1/2 cup rolled oats

- 1/2 cup milk (dairy or plant-based)

- 1 apple, diced

- 1 tablespoon honey or maple syrup

- 1/2 teaspoon ground cinnamon

• Walnuts for topping

Instructions:

1. In a saucepan, combine rolled oats, milk, diced apple, sweetener, and cinnamon.

2. Cook over medium heat until the oats are tender.

3. Pour into a bowl and top with walnuts.

4. Tropical Mango Coconut Oatmeal:

Ingredients:

• 1/2 cup rolled oats

• 1/2 cup coconut milk

• 1/2 cup diced mango

• 1 tablespoon shredded coconut

• 1 teaspoon chia seeds

• Pineapple chunks for topping

Instructions:

1. In a saucepan, cook rolled oats with coconut milk until creamy.

2. Stir in diced mango, shredded coconut, and chia seeds.

3. Cook for an additional 2-3 minutes.

4. Pour into a bowl and top with pineapple chunks.

5. Peanut Butter Banana Protein Oats:

Ingredients:

• 1/2 cup rolled oats

• 1/2 cup milk (dairy or plant-based)

• 1 ripe banana, sliced

• 1 tablespoon peanut butter

• 1 scoop protein powder (vanilla or chocolate)

• Sliced banana and a drizzle of peanut butter for topping

Instructions:

1. In a saucepan, combine rolled oats, milk, sliced banana, and peanut butter.

2. Cook over medium heat until the oats are tender.

3. Stir in the protein powder until well combined.

4. Pour into a bowl, top with sliced banana, and drizzle with additional peanut butter.

## Lunch and Dinner Recipes

Certainly! Here's a compilation of 20 lunch and dinner recipes with step-by-step instructions and ingredients:

1. Grilled Chicken Caesar Salad:

Ingredients:

• Grilled chicken breast

• Romaine lettuce

• Cherry tomatoes

• Croutons

• Parmesan cheese

• Caesar dressing

Instructions:

1. Grill chicken until fully cooked.

2. Chop romaine lettuce and halve cherry tomatoes.

3. Slice grilled chicken and toss with lettuce, tomatoes, croutons, and Parmesan.

4. Drizzle with Caesar dressing before serving.

2. Quinoa and Black Bean Bowl:

Ingredients:

• Cooked quinoa

• Black beans

• Corn kernels

• Diced tomatoes

• Avocado slices

• Lime wedges

Instructions:

1. Mix cooked quinoa, black beans, corn, and diced tomatoes.

2. Top with avocado slices.

3. Squeeze lime juice over the bowl before serving.

3. Teriyaki Salmon with Stir-Fried Vegetables:

Ingredients:

• Salmon fillets

• Teriyaki sauce

• Broccoli

• Bell peppers

• Carrots

• Soy sauce

Instructions:

1. Marinate salmon in teriyaki sauce.

2. Grill or bake until cooked through.

3. Stir-fry broccoli, bell peppers, and carrots with soy sauce.

4. Serve salmon over the stir-fried vegetables.

4. Lentil and Vegetable Stir-Fry:

Ingredients:

• Cooked lentils

• Mixed vegetables (bell peppers, broccoli, carrots)

• Soy sauce

• Garlic

• Ginger

• Sesame oil

Instructions:

1. Sauté cooked lentils and mixed vegetables in sesame oil.

2. Add minced garlic and ginger.

3. Drizzle with soy sauce and stir until heated through.

5. Shrimp and Asparagus Risotto:

Ingredients:

• Arborio rice

• Shrimp

• Asparagus

• Chicken broth

• White wine

• Parmesan cheese

Instructions:

1. Sauté shrimp and asparagus in olive oil.

2. Add Arborio rice and cook until translucent.

3. Pour in white wine and stir until absorbed.

4. Gradually add chicken broth while stirring until rice is creamy.

5. Stir in Parmesan cheese before serving.

6. Chickpea and Spinach Curry:

Ingredients:

• Chickpeas

• Fresh spinach

- Onion

- Garlic

- Curry spices (turmeric, cumin, coriander)

- Coconut milk

Instructions:

1. Sauté chopped onion and garlic in a pan.

2. Add curry spices and stir.

3. Pour in coconut milk and add chickpeas.

4. Simmer until chickpeas are tender, then stir in fresh spinach.

7. Caprese Quinoa Salad:

Ingredients:

- Cooked quinoa

- Cherry tomatoes

- Fresh mozzarella

- Basil leaves

- Balsamic glaze

Instructions:

1. Mix cooked quinoa with halved cherry tomatoes.

2. Add diced fresh mozzarella and torn basil leaves.

3. Drizzle with balsamic glaze before serving.

8. Turkey and Avocado Wrap:

Ingredients:

• Sliced turkey breast

• Whole-grain tortilla

• Avocado slices

• Lettuce

• Tomato

• Greek yogurt dressing

Instructions:

1. Layer turkey, avocado, lettuce, and tomato on a tortilla.

2. Drizzle with Greek yogurt dressing.

3. Roll into a wrap and serve.

9. Beef and Broccoli Stir-Fry:

Ingredients:

• Beef strips

• Broccoli florets

- Soy sauce

- Garlic

- Ginger

- Sesame seeds

Instructions:

1. Sauté beef strips until browned.

2. Add broccoli and stir-fry until tender.

3. Mix in minced garlic and ginger.

4. Drizzle with soy sauce and sprinkle sesame seeds.

10. Mediterranean Chickpea Salad:

Ingredients:

- Chickpeas

- Cucumber

- Cherry tomatoes

- Kalamata olives

- Feta cheese

- Olive oil and lemon dressing

Instructions:

1. Combine chickpeas, diced cucumber, halved cherry tomatoes, sliced olives, and crumbled feta.

2. Toss with olive oil and lemon dressing.

11. Baked Cod with Lemon Dill Sauce:

Ingredients:

• Cod fillets

• Lemon

• Fresh dill

• Olive oil

• Garlic

• Salt and pepper

Instructions:

1. Season cod with minced garlic, chopped dill, and lemon slices.

2. Drizzle with olive oil and bake until fish flakes.

3. Serve with a squeeze of lemon.

12. Quinoa and Vegetable Stuffed Bell Peppers:

Ingredients:

• Quinoa

• Bell peppers

• Black beans

• Corn

• Salsa

• Shredded cheese

Instructions:

1. Cook quinoa and mix with black beans, corn, and salsa.

2. Cut bell peppers in half and stuff with quinoa mixture.

3. Top with shredded cheese and bake until peppers are tender.

13. Thai Peanut Chicken Stir-Fry:

Ingredients:

• Chicken breast strips

• Broccoli

• Bell peppers

• Carrots

• Peanut sauce

• Rice noodles

Instructions:

1. Stir-fry chicken until cooked.

2. Add broccoli, bell peppers, and julienned carrots.

3. Mix in peanut sauce and serve over cooked rice noodles.

14. Veggie and Lentil Curry:

Ingredients:

• Lentils

• Mixed vegetables (zucchini, bell peppers, carrots)

• Coconut milk

• Curry spices (cumin, coriander, turmeric)

• Basmati rice

Instructions:

1. Cook lentils and set aside.

2. Sauté mixed vegetables in a pan.

3. Stir in coconut milk and curry spices.

4. Add cooked lentils and simmer until heated through.

5. Serve over basmati rice.

15. Baked Chicken Thighs with Roasted Brussels Sprouts:

Ingredients:

• Chicken thighs

• Brussels sprouts

• Olive oil

• Garlic

• Paprika

• Salt and pepper

Instructions:

1. Season chicken thighs with minced garlic, paprika, salt, and pepper.

2. Arrange chicken on a baking sheet with halved Brussels sprouts.

3. Drizzle with olive oil and bake until chicken is golden.

16. Mediterranean Quinoa Stuffed Peppers:

Ingredients:

• Quinoa

• Cherry tomatoes

• Cucumber

• Red onion

• Feta cheese

• Olive oil and balsamic vinegar

Instructions:

1. Cook quinoa and let it cool.

2. Mix quinoa with halved cherry tomatoes, diced cucumber, red onion, and crumbled feta.

3. Drizzle with olive oil and balsamic vinegar.

4. Stuff the mixture into halved bell peppers.

17. Sweet Potato and Black Bean Quesadillas:

Ingredients:

• Sweet potatoes, roasted and mashed

• Black beans

• Whole-grain tortillas

• Cumin and chili powder

• Shredded cheese

• Guacamole for serving

Instructions:

1. Mash roasted sweet potatoes and mix with black beans, cumin, and chili powder.

2. Spread the mixture on a tortilla, sprinkle with cheese, and top with another tortilla.

3. Cook on a griddle until cheese melts.

4. Serve with guacamole.

18. Lemon Garlic Shrimp Pasta:

Ingredients:

• Shrimp

• Linguine pasta

• Olive oil

• Garlic

• Lemon zest and juice

• Parsley

• Parmesan cheese

Instructions:

1. Cook linguine according to package instructions.

2. Sauté shrimp in olive oil with minced garlic until pink.

3. Toss cooked pasta with shrimp, lemon zest, lemon juice, chopped parsley, and Parmesan.

19. Turkey and Quinoa Bowl:

Ingredients:

• Ground turkey

• Cooked quinoa

• Black beans

• Corn

• Salsa

• Avocado slices

Instructions:

1. Cook ground turkey until browned.

2. Mix with cooked quinoa, black beans, corn, and salsa.

3. Top with avocado slices.

20. Pesto Zucchini Noodles with Cherry Tomatoes:

Ingredients:

• Zucchini noodles

• Pesto sauce

• Cherry tomatoes, halved

• Pine nuts

• Parmesan cheese

Instructions:

1. Sauté zucchini noodles in a pan until tender.

2. Toss with pesto sauce and halved cherry tomatoes.

3. Top with pine nuts and Parmesan before serving.

## Snacks and Quick Bites

Certainly! Here are 10 tasty snacks and quick bites with step-by-step instructions and ingredients:

1. Guacamole and Whole Wheat Pita Chips:

Ingredients:

• Ripe avocados

• Diced tomatoes

• Red onion

• Cilantro

• Lime juice

• Whole wheat pita bread

Instructions:

1. Mash avocados and mix with diced tomatoes, finely chopped red onion, cilantro, and lime juice.

2. Toast whole wheat pita bread and cut it into triangles.

3. Dip pita chips into guacamole and enjoy!

2. Greek Yogurt Parfait with Berries:

Ingredients:

• Greek yogurt

• Mixed berries (strawberries, blueberries, raspberries)

• Granola

• Honey

Instructions:

1. Layer Greek yogurt in a glass or bowl.

2. Add mixed berries and granola.

3. Drizzle with honey before serving.

3. Hummus and Vegetable Sticks:

Ingredients:

• Hummus

• Carrot sticks

• Cucumber slices

• Bell pepper strips

Instructions:

1. Arrange vegetable sticks on a plate.

2. Dip into your favorite hummus.

4. Caprese Skewers:

Ingredients:

• Cherry tomatoes

• Mozzarella balls

• Fresh basil leaves

• Balsamic glaze

Instructions:

1. Thread cherry tomatoes, mozzarella balls, and fresh basil leaves onto skewers.

2. Drizzle with balsamic glaze before serving.

5. Cottage Cheese and Pineapple Bowls:

Ingredients:

• Cottage cheese

• Pineapple chunks

• Chopped mint (optional)

Instructions:

1. Scoop cottage cheese into bowls.

2. Top with pineapple chunks and garnish with chopped mint.

6. Almond Butter and Banana Sandwiches:

Ingredients:

- Whole grain bread

- Almond butter

- Sliced bananas

Instructions:

1. Spread almond butter on whole grain bread slices.

2. Add sliced bananas between the slices to make sandwiches.

7. Roasted Chickpeas:

Ingredients:

- Canned chickpeas, drained

- Olive oil

- Paprika

- Garlic powder

- Salt

Instructions:

1. Toss chickpeas with olive oil, paprika, garlic powder, and salt.

2. Roast in the oven until crispy.

8. Rice Cake with Avocado and Cherry Tomatoes:

Ingredients:

• Rice cakes

• Ripe avocado

• Cherry tomatoes, halved

• Salt and pepper

Instructions:

1. Spread mashed avocado on rice cakes.

2. Top with halved cherry tomatoes and season with salt and pepper.

9. Apple Slices with Nut Butter:

Ingredients:

• Apple, sliced

• Almond or peanut butter

Instructions:

1. Spread nut butter on apple slices.

2. Enjoy this simple and satisfying snack.

10. Trail Mix with Nuts and Dried Fruits:

Ingredients:

• Mixed nuts (almonds, walnuts, cashews)

• Dried fruits (raisins, cranberries)

• Dark chocolate chunks

Instructions:

1. Combine mixed nuts, dried fruits, and dark chocolate chunks in a bowl.

2. Portion into small snack bags for a convenient on-the-go option.

## Final Thoughts

As you embark on your culinary journey with this bodybuilding diet cookbook, keep in mind the importance of nourishing your body with balanced and nutritious meals. Each recipe is crafted to support your fitness goals and provide the energy needed for your workouts. Remember to listen to your body, make adjustments as needed, and enjoy the process of preparing and savoring these delicious meals.

Whether you're fueling up before a workout, recovering after an intense session, or simply indulging in a satisfying and healthy meal, these recipes are designed to cater to your body's nutritional requirements. Feel free to explore additional variations, swap ingredients based on your preferences, and get creative in the kitchen.

Consistency is key in both your diet and exercise routine. Stay committed to your fitness journey, and let this cookbook be a helpful companion along the way. Here's to achieving your bodybuilding goals, one nutritious and flavorful meal at a time!

Happy cooking and best of luck on your fitness journey!